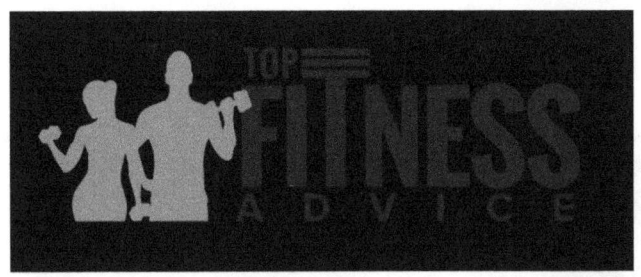

WEIGHT LOSS HACKS

15+ Powerful Hacks That Can Help Boost Your Metabolism And Lead To Weight Loss While You Sleep (Eat Your Way To Skinny)

LINDA WESTWOOD

First published in 2015 by Venture Ink Publishing

Copyright © Top Fitness Advice 2019

All rights reserved.

No part of this book may be reproduced in any form without permission in writing from the author. No part of this publication may be reproduced or transmitted in any form or by any means, mechanic, electronic, photocopying, recording, by any storage or retrieval system, or transmitted by email without the permission in writing from the author and publisher.

Requests to the publisher for permission should be addressed to publishing@ventureink.co

For more information about the contents of this book or questions to the author, please contact Linda Westwood at linda@topfitnessadvice.com

Disclaimer

This book provides wellness management information in an informative and educational manner only, with information that is general in nature and that is not specific to you, the reader. The contents of this book are intended to assist you and other readers in your personal wellness efforts. Consult your physician regarding the applicability of any information provided in this book to you.

Nothing in this book should be construed as personal advice or diagnosis, and must not be used in this manner. The information provided about conditions is general in nature. This information does not cover all possible uses, actions, precautions, side-effects, or interactions of medicines, or medical procedures. The information in this book should not be considered as complete and does not cover all diseases, ailments, physical conditions, or their treatment.

You should consult with your physician before beginning any exercise, weight loss, or health care program. This book should not be used in place of a call or visit to a competent health-care professional. You should consult a health care professional before adopting any of the suggestions in this book or before drawing inferences from it.

Any decision regarding treatment and medication for your condition should be made with the advice and consultation of a qualified health care professional. If you have, or suspect you have, a health-care problem, then you should immediately contact a qualified health care professional for treatment.

No Warranties: The author and publisher don't guarantee or warrant the quality, accuracy, completeness, timeliness, appropriateness or suitability of the information in this book, or of any product or services referenced in this book.

The information in this book is provided on an "as is" basis and the author and publisher make no representations or warranties of any kind with respect to this information. This book may contain inaccuracies, typographical errors, or other errors.

Liability Disclaimer: The publisher, author, and other parties involved in the creation, production, provision of information, or delivery of this book specifically disclaim any responsibility, and shall not be held liable for any damages, claims, injuries, losses, liabilities, costs, or obligations including any direct, indirect, special, incidental, or consequences damages (collectively known as "Damages") whatsoever and howsoever caused, arising out of, or in connection with the use or misuse of the site and the information contained within it, whether such Damages arise in contract, tort, negligence, equity, statute law, or by way of other legal theory.

Table of Contents

Disclaimer	3
Who is this book for?	9
What will this book teach you?	11
9-Step System to Lose Weight While You Sleep	13
Step 1: Always Be Eating	19
Step 2: Binge Drink Your Fat Away	25
Step 3: Start Eating Fat Burning Foods	31
Step 4: Stop Working Out So Much	37
Step 5: The Secrets to Burning Fat While You Sleep	43
Step 6: Take Your Fat Burning to The Next Level	49
Step 7: Insulin Is Your Enemy	55
Step 8: Eat Junk Food & Lose Weight	61
Step 9: Boost Your Fat Burning TODAY!	65
Don't Forget This!	71
The PROVEN & EFFECTIVE Way to Boost Your Metabolism Permanently	73
Understanding Your Metabolism	75

Factors That Determine Your Metabolic Rate	77
Fat Burning and Body Toning Foods	83
Tips on How to Speed Up Your Basal Metabolic Rate	91
Nutrition	101
Factors That May Slow Down Metabolism	105
Final Words	113

Would you prefer to listen to my book, rather than read it?

Download the audiobook version for free!

If you go to the special link below and sign up to Audible as a new customer, you can get the audiobook version of my book completely free.

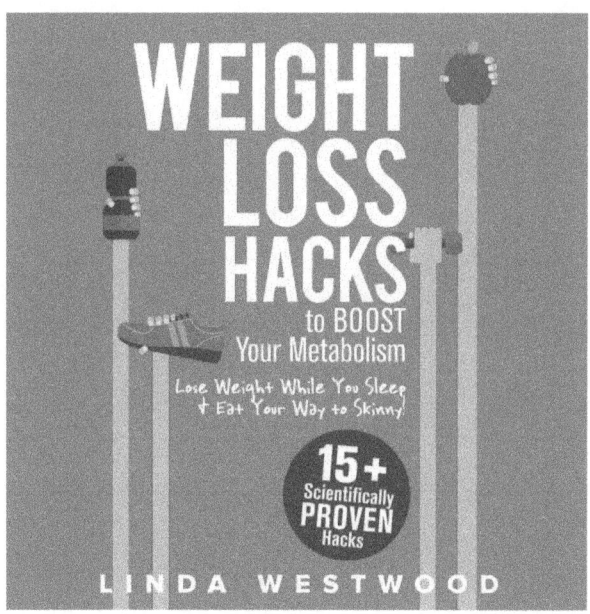

Go here to get your audiobook version for free:

TopFitnessAdvice.com/go/WeightHacks

Who is this book for?

Are you finding it hard to lose weight and keep it off?

Do you hate working out so much and seeing NO results?

Do you wish you could burn fat *while you sleep* and shed sizes *without even trying?*

Do you want to learn some POWERFUL weight loss hacks that ACTUALLY WORK?

Then this book is for you!

I am going to share with you two things: a 9-step system that, when applied, will help you melt your fat while you sleep, AND a comprehensive nutritional strategy that you can implement to boost your metabolism and burn more fat all day, every day.

The information in this book is comprehensive and you will be able to apply it immediately into your life because there are action plans and step-by-step instructions included!

Whether you're a complete beginner, or someone who works out regularly, it doesn't matter!

If this sounds like it could help you, keep reading...

What will this book teach you?

Inside this book, I will teach you in great detail how you can start melting *MORE* fat than ever before, even while you sleep!

How?

Firstly, because you're going to learn every part of the 9-step system that will elevate your metabolic rate to a point where your body is melting its own fat 24/7!

In each of the steps, not only will you learn what you need to implement in your life, and why you need to implement it – but also HOW you can start doing it *immediately!*

This 9-step system is completely unique and contains steps that have never before been put together. It *really* does work!

Secondly, you will also learn the most effective changes you can make to your diet and nutrition to MAXIMISE and BOOST your metabolism so your fat begins to melt and the pounds fall off automatically without you having to do any extra work!

Both these systems are great and really do work - however...

For the best results, you *must* be sure to implement it in your life.

Unfortunately, too many people will read this system and do absolutely nothing about it – so I strongly urge you to take action immediately!

9-Step System to Lose Weight While You Sleep

What You Need to Know Before You Begin

The whole philosophy behind eating food to lose weight has to do with your metabolism.

If you can understand the terms "metabolism" and "metabolic rate," then you will be on your way to burning fat with food in no time.

What is the Metabolism?

The metabolism describes a series of chemical reactions within the cells of the body. These chemical reactions occur when food passes through our digestive system and converts the nutrients from the food into energy for the body.

We are all born with a metabolism. It stays with us throughout our entire lives until we are dead. It is what keeps us moving, growing and thinking.

The chemical reactions in our cells are controlled by the proteins in our body. Each chemical reaction is responsible for a different function of the body. That is why we have thousands of chemical reactions happening in our body at the same time.

Energy is measured in units that are called "calories." When you look at the nutritional label on food, you will find how many calories that food has per serving. These calories should be thought of as units of energy.

What is the Metabolic Rate?

The metabolic rate is the rate at which calories are burned in the body to produce energy; we will look at this rate at rest (for simplicity).

The metabolic rate is often referred to by doctors and health experts as the BMR, which stands for basal metabolic rate.

It is important to know your BMR because it will help you determine how much energy you burn during your sleep and how many calories you need to consume from your food intake.

A person with a low BMR will burn fewer calories while they are asleep and someone with a high BMR will burn more calories.

If a person with low BMR consumes more calories than they burn, then these excess calories will turn to fat.

People with high BMRs normally don't have a problem losing weight.

It is those with low BMRs that struggle the most with gaining weight and then trying to lose it. That is why these people need to focus on ways to boost their metabolic rate. That way they can burn more calories during their sleep than they normally would.

The important thing to remember is that our metabolisms burn calories regardless of whether or not we exercise.

The only difference is people who exercise will boost their metabolic rates even higher and lose more weight while they sleep, but we will get into that later on in this book.

The 9-Step System Solution

You now know how the metabolic rate coincides with gaining weight and losing weight.

This book features a 9-step system that will teach you how to successfully boost your metabolic rate, so you can finally lose weight once and for all.

The 9 steps in this book should be followed in order.

Start from the very first step and slowly progress to the next step after a couple of days. You will find the steps get harder as you progress, but don't give up!

If you implement the 9-step system into your daily lifestyle, then you should see a significant boost in your metabolic rate.

This will turn your body into a fat burning machine.

Discover Scientifically-Proven "Shortcuts" & "Hacks" to Lose Weight FASTER (With Very Little Effort)

For this month only, you can get Linda's best-selling & most popular book absolutely free – *Weight Loss Secrets You NEED to Know*.

Get Your FREE Copy Here:
TopFitnessAdvice.com/Bonus

Discover scientifically-proven tips to help you lose weight faster and easier than ever before. With this book, readers were able to improve their weight loss results and fitness levels. So, it's highly recommended that you get this book, especially while it's free!

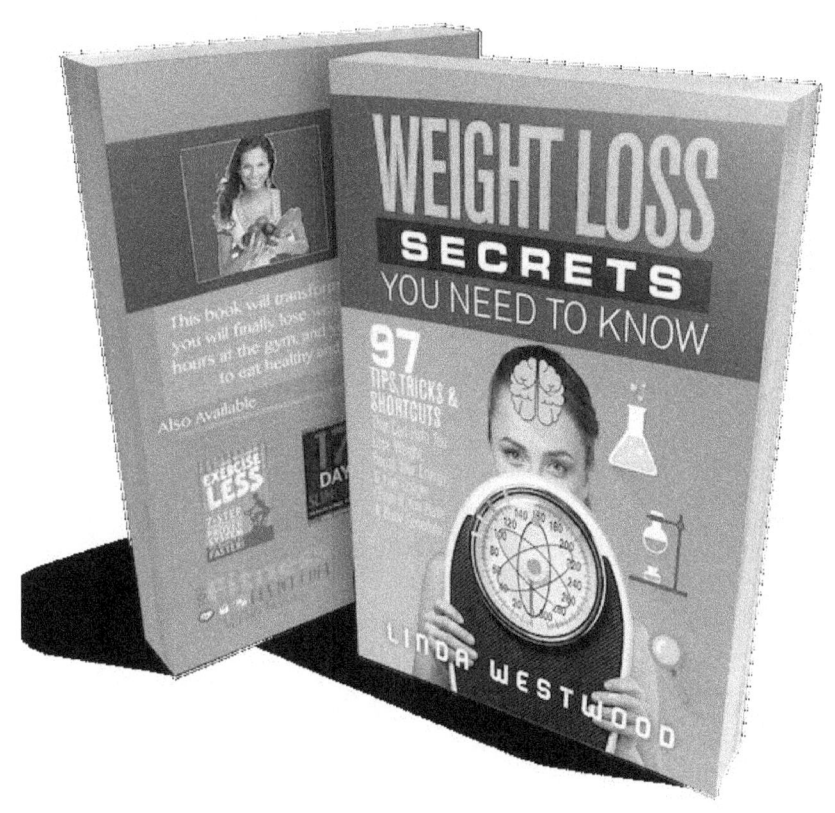

Get Your FREE Copy Here:
TopFitnessAdvice.com/Bonus

Step 1

Always Be Eating

When people hear for the first time that the secret to losing weight is eating more food, they may think it's crazy.

But the truth is that eating frequently throughout the day will increase your metabolic rate, which will in turn cause you to burn fat and lose weight.

Breakfast is Always Important

While growing up, we have all heard adults tell us that breakfast is the most important meal of the day.

They are right because our body just got through sleeping for eight hours, and during those eight hours we did not eat anything.

As soon as you wake up in the morning, you should have something to eat in order to get your metabolism jump started to start the day.

People often complain about not being hungry in the morning, despite not eating for eight hours.

You can always eat something small, like Greek yogurt or a banana, to give you a healthy start to your day.

Six Meals per Day

If you ask any nutritionist, personal trainer or health expert, they will all agree that eating six small meals per day is better than eating three bigger sized meals per day.

The metabolism is like a burning fireplace. To keep the fire going, you have to periodically put more wood into the fire or else the fire will stop burning.

In the case of eating food, if you eat three meals per day then you are likely waiting six hours in between meals.

Then after dinner, you won't be eating anything until breakfast the next day. This could be almost 12 hours of not eating anything, which is too long for the metabolism.

Eight hours should be the biggest gap of the day.

When you eat six meals per day, you are typically eating a small meal every 3 hours. Not only that, but it will keep your blood sugar steady as well. That way you don't over stuff yourself with food, which will allow you to be hungry in 3 hours.

If you eat a large meal then you won't be hungry for a long time because there is an abundance of food trying to pass through your digestive system. This will still slow down your metabolism though, which will then cause all the excess calories to get stored as fat on your body instead of getting burned for energy.

You ever noticed how sluggish and bloated you feel after eating a big meal, like at a buffet?

This is the result of too many calories.

But if you eat a small meal with just enough calories to burn into energy, then your body won't be storing any excess calories as fat.

This will give you a nice natural boost of energy that you need to make it through your day.

How do I determine a small meal versus a large meal?

Small meals are normally calculated by the amount of recommended calories you should have in each meal. To figure this out, you need to first know your BMR.

Get onto Google and search for BMR calculators. You will find dozens of them listed in the search results.

Pick a calculator and then fill in the calculation requirements. They will ask for your weight, height, age and gender.

The results will give you the total calories you need per day in order to get the precise amount of energy for your body to function properly.

Once you figure this out, divide the BMR by six (which represents the number of meals you will need per day).

For example, let's say you are a male who is six feet tall and weighs 240 pounds. Your BMR will be 2,082 calories per day.

Now divide 2,082 by 6, and you get 347.

This means you need 347 calories per meal.

This may seem like a lot, but once you start studying nutritional labels you will quickly learn how easy it is to consume 347 calories.

You could easily get this from just eating one slice of whole wheat toast and an apple.

Why Six Meals? Why Every 3 Hours?

These are all good questions that newcomers always ask when they hear about the six-meal diet. There are actually scientific reasons as to why you need to eat six meals per day; 1 every 3 hours.

After you go 3 hours without having any food in your system, this is when your blood sugar begins to fall.

At this point, you will start to feel hungry because your body will almost be finished digesting all the food you ate earlier.

Then after 4 hours, it will be completely finished digesting the food. Four hours is the absolute longest you should wait to eat.

If you make it to the 5 hour mark or beyond without eating any food, your blood sugar will tumble. This will make you want to grab any food you see nearby and overeat.

A good example of this is with people who work long hours and don't get a chance to eat very often.

After the lunch break at 12 noon, they won't get another chance to eat until they get out of work at 5.

By this time, they will feel compelled to drive by the local fast food joint because they are so hungry. This is why so many people are overweight.

What You Eat Is Always Important

You may wonder if eating six meals of junk food per day is better than eating three meals of healthy food per day.

The answer is no.

Do not think because you are boosting your metabolism with six meals that it gives you the right to eat whatever you want. You still have to be responsible with your food choices. This means eating natural foods whenever possible.

If you were to eat three meals of healthy food, you would not lose much weight but at least you would be maintaining a healthy heart and a number of other benefits.

But still, why settle for the bare minimum? Why not eat six meals of healthy food per day? Then you can burn fat and keep your body healthy at the same time. The best part is that healthy food is easy to prepare and you can eat it quickly.

Step 2

Binge Drink Your Fat Away

Yes!

I want you to binge drink…

Binge drink water!

There are two types of drinks in this world. There are drinks that nourish your body and help to burn fat and there are drinks that add fat to your body.

The drinks that add fat are all those processed drinks you see in stores. These are the primarily the fruit juices, sodas and flavored milks.

While flavored milk and fruit juices may have some minor health benefits, they are still loaded with added sugars and calories.

If you drink a drink with calories in it, then it is very easy to add on extra weight because you will keep on drinking without feeling full. That is why you should only get your calories from food, not drinks.

Water is the Best Drink

Water will always be the best beverage you can ever drink. It is natural for our bodies and provides a variety of health benefits.

Water can help people lose weight.

The more water you drink, the faster you speed up the digestion of the foods you have eaten. This allows you to burn calories faster and feel more energetic in the process.

People who do not drink water become dehydrated. Dehydration will cause your bodily organs to work harder in order to perform their most basic functions.

When this happens, the body will store water in its fat cells, which increases the size of the cells and makes you become fatter.

By hydrating your body with water, it will not have to store water in the fat cells. This will decrease the size of the cells and actually make you lose fat.

Plus, your internal organs will be able to function better and put less strain on your body.

To effectively hydrate your body, it is recommended that you drink eight glasses of water per day, but preferably more.

Try to take sips of water after every bite of your food. That will help your digestive system process it faster, as well as help you feel fuller quicker (leading to less calories eaten).

You can also drink water in between meals without any problem because water has zero calories. Therefore, you will never get fat from drinking water.

Use water as a replacement for binging on junk food snacks, like potato chips and chocolate bars. Sometimes when our bodies are thirsty we often mistake this thirst for hunger. By drinking water as a snack, you will lose those hunger pains.

Psychological Health from Water

Studies have shown that dehydrated people have weaker cognitive functions than those who hydrate themselves with water.

People who are thirsty cannot concentrate on what is in front of them because they are mentally distracted by their thirst. They will eventually get light headed from being dehydrated as well.

Hydrated people feel more energetic and can think clearly. Some even have better memory as a result of drinking more water.

Water Does Not Work Miracles

People who want to lose weight often get excited when they hear about a technique that lets them burn fat, like drinking lots of water.

It is true that water can help you lose weight and function better, but it cannot do everything by itself. In other words, you still have to maintain a healthy diet in order to lose the weight.

For example, if you eat cheeseburgers from the local fast food joint and then just replace your soda with water, you are not going to lose much weight because you are still eating the cheeseburgers.

You have to eat healthy foods and drink water at the same time. This will allow you to lose more weight and increase the health of your other internal organs.

Green Tea

Green tea is a great alternative to water and will provide you with lots of antioxidants, which will clean out your body of toxins and free radicals.

Studies have shown green tea can help people lose weight if they consume at least 2-3 cups of green tea per day. It will flush away fat and keep your body healthy at the same time.

Think about drinking green tea with a few of your other meals. It will help boost your metabolism while eating, which will allow you to absorb more energy from the foods you are eating.

Cranberry Water

Cranberry water is a unique drink that not a lot of people know about. It is basically a combination of water and cranberry juice, which will flush fat out of your body a lot faster than just drinking one of the two liquids.

The high amounts of organic acids in the cranberry juice will be responsible for dissolving a majority of the fatty deposits in your body. By adding water to it, the acids make contact with the deposits faster.

Grapefruit Juice

Grapefruit is a natural type of fruit juice with no added sugars or preservatives. More importantly, it contains high levels of Vitamin C and helps support a healthy liver.

In case you did not know, the liver is responsible for detoxifying your body of free radicals and other dangerous toxins that enter your body from food consumption. So, if you have a healthy liver, it will continue to metabolize and detoxify your body at a rapid rate.

No Substitutes

When it comes to drinking something healthy, like water, people often find ways around drinking the pure natural spring water. Instead, they will replace it with something processed or modified.

Please note that flavored water and carbonated water are not the waters you should be drinking. These have added ingredients that take away the "natural" element you want in your water.

Water with added minerals is also something to watch out for. Although not totally bad, this water is known to have an abundance of minerals. This can add pressure to the kidneys and cause a variety of health problems in the long run.

In order to verify if your water is pure or not, just look at the ingredients on the nutritional label. If there is any ingredient other than water, then it has been modified and you should not drink it.

Step 3

Start Eating Fat Burning Foods

You have probably seen plenty of metabolism boosting supplements advertised on television and the internet.

However, these supplements are a waste of money because you can get the metabolic boost much faster and more naturally from simply eating the right foods.

The secret to increasing your metabolic rate from the food you eat is by studying the vitamins and nutrients that are in your food.

Some of the best nutrients for burning food are Complex 'B' Vitamins, Iron, L-carnitine amino acid, and chitosan; just to name a few. So, all you have to do is find foods with these nutrients in them.

Best Fat Burning Nutrients

- **L-carnitine** – Both red meat and lean meats contain the L-carnitine amino acid, which will increase the fat burning process if taken before an exercise routine.

    If you are lifting weights, then you will also be glad to get an extra dose of protein from the meats as well. The meats you can eat include steak, chicken, seafood, pork and even liver.

- **Chitosan** – Chitosan is a special sugar that is extracted from the outside shells of lobster, crab, and shrimp. Doctors often prescribe supplements of chitosan to patients who suffer from high cholesterol, obesity and kidney problems.

  For those simply looking to lose weight before they get to this point, you can simply eat the foods that contain chitosan in them.

  When ingested in your body, it works to block the absorption of cholesterol and dietary fat. This is how it keeps you from gaining weight.

- **Vitamin B** – There are many complex Vitamin B foods out there which will boost your metabolic rate. These foods include leafy green vegetables, lentils, whole grains, and almonds.

  The main function of B vitamins is to metabolize the fats, carbohydrates and proteins from the food in order to utilize the energy contained in them for the body.

- **Iron** – Iron is responsible for carrying oxygen to the muscles of your body, which allows them to burn off fat. Without iron, you will have a low metabolic rate and this will result in having little energy. Some great sources of iron include shellfish, spinach, beans and lean meats.

- **Fiber** – Fiber is crucial for processing food properly in your digestive system. Some of the best fiber foods are oatmeal and beans.

  It is recommended that you have oatmeal after you first wake up in the morning. Then you won't feel compelled to stop off from a doughnut or McMuffin from any fast food drive-thru.

Food Substitutions

If you have a problem with excess fat on your body then you are likely eating junk foods or fewer meals, which slows down your metabolic rate.

The ability to break the habit of eating bad foods can almost be as hard as beating a drug addiction. In fact, it can be worse because we see junk foods advertised and eaten everywhere we go. So, the temptation is always going to be there.

The best way to go about switching up your foods in order to boost your metabolic rate is to start slow and make minor substitutions in your food choices.

For example, if you typically like to snack on junk foods from the vending machine at work, like potato chips, then try to find an alternative snack that is healthier.

A bag of almonds is a great alternative because they are small and can easily be eaten from a bag. Not only that, but they don't cause a mess on your hands like potato chip grease does.

Now when it comes to bigger meals, you just need to pay attention to your assortment of foods. Do not choose processed or frozen boxed foods under any circumstances, even if they contain the nutrients mentioned above.

Processed foods have other added ingredients, like sodium and salt, which make you retain water. This will give you a bloated look that you don't want to have.

So, if you like to have a chicken TV dinner, try replacing that with a chicken breast from the deli at the supermarket instead. Then for a side dish, use green vegetables and beans.

With frequent meals like this, your metabolic rate will be through the roof. This, of course, will mean an increase in fat loss.

Moderate Coffee Consumption is Good

When you wake up in the morning and have your cup of coffee, you are actually doing more than giving yourself a boost of energy. You are speeding up your heart rate, which in turn gives your metabolic rate a boost as well.

You probably already know why coffee gives you a boost. It is because of the caffeine that is in coffee.

If you work out at the gym or perform any type of exercise, you may want to take coffee before you start the physical activity.

This will give you the boost you need to excel better while you are working out. Not only that, but it will push your metabolic rate even higher than it already is.

Caffeine can be an asset to helping you lose weight, but do not abuse it. Caffeine can become an addiction if you become too dependent on it for energy.

Weightlifters often take pre-workout supplements that have an unusually high amount of caffeine in them. You should avoid getting caffeine from a pre-workout supplement because it could boost your heart rate up to the point where it could give you a heart attack.

Eating before Sleep

You will hear a lot of conflicting advice about how close to bedtime you should be eating your meals.

Some people will tell you not to eat within 3 hours of going to sleep because a full stomach will turn your food into fat and not absorb energy. For those eating three meals of unhealthy foods every night, this may be true.

If you stick to six small meals per day and eat the foods mentioned in this chapter, it does not matter how close to bedtime you eat. In fact, it is actually better to eat a small meal before going to sleep.

That way you won't get hungry in the middle of the night and start binging on junk foods.

Don't forget you won't be eating for the next eight hours, so you should have something in your belly before the lights go out. Therefore, keep eating every three hours and do not starve yourself before bedtime.

I hope that you are enjoying this book so far, and if you could spare 30 seconds, I would greatly appreciate you leaving a review on Amazon.com.

Step 4

Stop Working Out So Much

There are many misconceptions out there about how much time you need to spend in the gym while working out. The typical person will assume that more time in the gym will mean more calories burned. This is not the case.

All you will end up doing is physically exert yourself, which will decrease the intensity of your workout. Then you will be too tired to get anything done.

It is better to exercise with high intensity for a short period of time and then take a rest. If you do, then your metabolic rate will stay boosted as you continue to fuel it with healthy small meals like previous discussed.

Cardiovascular Exercise & Fat Burning

Doctors may tell their overweight patients to try walking in order to lose weight, but this may not always be the case (depending on the health of the patient's heart).

There is something called high intensity interval training, or HIIT, which is basically a routine where you perform high intensity cardiovascular workouts in short periods of time. Cardiovascular workouts are basically any form of exercise that consistently gets your heart rate up. The most famous exercises like this are walking, jogging, running, biking and swimming.

The greatest intensity workout will be running as fast as you can in short intervals. For example, if you go on the treadmill then warm up with a 4-mph jog. After two minutes, then switch to a 7-mph run. Do this for another two minutes and then repeat. Keep going like this for at least 10-20 minutes and then you can stop.

By the time you are done with all these intervals, your metabolic rate will be very high. In fact, it will be so high that you will continue to burn calories long after you have stopped working out!

Weight Lifting & Fat Burning

People who lift weights don't typically think about the fat they are burning. They just think about getting big muscles that rip through their skin.

What many weightlifters don't think about is how lifting weights actually increases their heart rate and metabolic rate. But, they have to lift a certain way to really get the metabolic boost they are looking for.

People who lift really heavy weights for 3-4 repetitions and then take a 2-minute rest will not have much of a metabolic boost. Instead, those who lift lighter weights for 8-12 repetitions and take 30 second breaks will have a much higher boost.

You have to understand that weightlifting is not about lifting super heavy weights to get big muscles.

In fact, you can still get big muscles by lifting lighter weights with more repetitions. Not only does this turn you into a fat burning machine that will define your muscles, but it allows you to keep proper form and prevents you from getting injured.

It is also a good idea to confuse your muscles every couple of weeks by going back to heavy weights. After you have burned lots of calories with your lightweight workouts, try one week of heavy weight workouts in order to increase your muscle size.

This muscle increase will end up burning more calories while you are resting because this is when your body repairs itself. As your muscles are getting rebuilt, your metabolic rate is increasing as well.

Just remember to keep the rest periods to a minimum in between sets. That way, the workout will stay intense, which will keep your metabolic rate high after the workout.

Resistance Training

When you build muscle, you are burning more calories.

The bigger your muscles are, the more fat you are going to burn.

Resistance training is a great weightlifting technique that builds muscle and boosts the metabolism. It will cause you to boost your metabolism for at least 35 hours straight after a workout.

A typical resistance training routine could be as follows:

DAY ONE: Barbell Bench Press (3 Sets), Lat Pull Downs (3 Sets)

DAY TWO: Bicep Curls (4 Sets), Tricep Bench Dips (4 Sets)

DAY THREE: Front Deltoid Raises (3 Sets), Leg Squats (2 Sets)

You could mix about 10 minutes of cardiovascular exercise on those days if you don't feel tired after the weight workouts. But if you are using the right amount of weight, then you should be tired.

This is when you should stop, so the body can enter its recovery mode.

Things to Remember

If you learn anything from this chapter, it should be this: Focus on burning fat after your workout, not during your workout.

If fat melted off during exercise, then everybody would walk out of the gym looking lean with a six-pack.

The reason why people don't burn fat during exercise is because the body burns carbohydrates (broken down into glucose) to use as its fuel source for energy.

If the workout is intense enough, the glucose will get used up. You will notice this when you start to feel tired and exhausted. At this point, you should stop working out.

Once you stop working out, your body will begin burning fat in order to recover because there are no more stored glucose left.

This is why people who overindulge in carbohydrates before and after a workout will not lose weight because the body will keep burning the carbohydrates and not the fat.

But in order for the metabolic rate to start burning fat, it needs to get into a resting period of recovery. If you keep pushing your workouts to longer than an hour, you won't be able to keep up the intensity you once had before because you will be out of energy.

Then you could risk other health issues, like heart attack or maybe even a decrease in muscle size.

Step 5

The Secrets to Burning Fat While You Sleep

There are no magic pills or weight loss products that are going to shred your body fat while you sleep. Do not believe what any "expert" from an infomercial tells you because they are just trying to sell you their product and will say anything to do so.

This does not mean there aren't secrets to burning fat while you sleep, because there are. You just have to know these true secrets and separate them from the untrue ones.

Get Enough Sleep

The first thing you should know about burning fat while you sleep is that you actually have to get an adequate amount of sleep. Don't think that you can just nap for 3 hours and be fully recovered for the next day.

The body needs at least 8 hours of sleep each night in order to effectively metabolize the body of any excess fats. So if you only sleep for 3 hours, then your metabolism won't be done burning fat from your body. This will cause your body to retain this fat instead.

Sleep deprivation adds a lot of stress to your body. There are two hormones in the body that regulate a person's sensations of feeling hungry and full. These are called ghrelin and leptin.

If you do not get enough sleep, these hormones will make you think you are hungry when you really aren't. Then you will overeat and gain more weight from thinking you are still hungry.

So, make sure you get enough sleep so these hormones can function properly and accurately tell you when you are truly hungry. If you have trouble getting to sleep, avoid having caffeine at nighttime or anything that might keep you awake.

If you live in a noisy environment, use earplugs to get silence at night. Whatever it takes to get a good night's sleep will be well worth it.

Eating the Right Foods

This goes back to the previous chapter where we talked about eating healthy foods and six small meals per day.

The foods we eat throughout the day and before we go to sleep play a crucial role in whether or not we get a good night's sleep. Make sure you are eating your six small meals of healthy foods throughout the day. Then by the time you go to sleep, your metabolic rate will be on fire.

If you were to eat a huge meal before going to sleep, you would be up all night feeling bloated and enduring stomach cramps. Then you'd have to periodically go to the bathroom. By the time you are ready to finally get some sleep, it will be the next morning and you will already have to start your day.

If you drink green tea before going to sleep, it will increase your fat oxidation and metabolic rate considerably because of its thermogenic properties. Green tea is also low in calories and contains less caffeine than a cup of coffee. Best of all, green tea has antioxidants to clean your body of free radicals and toxins.

As for your main foods, you want to incorporate whole grains and dairy products. Whole grains contain complex carbohydrates and fiber that will improve your body's metabolic functions.

Whole grains can be found in whole wheat, oatmeal, quinoa and brown rice. If you are not lactose intolerant, then the casein in cottage cheese and milk will help you lose fat while you sleep as well.

Resistance Training

Weight exercises might seem strange to do before going to sleep, but they are actually the best time to do them (now, I don't mean precisely before you sleep – rather, at some point in the evening, a few hours before sleeping).

Since resistance training exercises boost your metabolism, doing them in the evening will keep your metabolic rate very high throughout the night. That means you will be burning extra fat while you sleep. Resistance training before bedtime doesn't necessarily mean going to the gym and benching 225 pounds for a chest workout.

Instead, you could do pushups on the floor for chest or lunges for buttocks. Any resistance exercise that you can do in your room or home is suitable. Many people use exercise bands to get their resistance training at home. They can help you simulate lighter versions of exercises like squats, military presses, and bicep curls.

Cardiovascular Exercises

You already know that cardiovascular exercises such as running, walking and jogging are great ways to boost your metabolism and burn fat. That is why you need to do these exercises at nighttime as well.

Like with the resistance training, you don't have to do high intensity cardiovascular exercise before going to sleep. Just take a walk outside for 20 minutes or go on the treadmill if you have one. You could also do jumping jacks if you have no other options.

All you have to remember is to get your heart rate up with low intensity cardiovascular exercises. This will not only boost your metabolic rate, but it will put you in a state of relaxation so you can get a good night's sleep.

Supplements

After you have exhausted the diet and exercise options for boosting your metabolism, you could always go further with it by integrating supplements into your routine. Supplements should never replace diet and exercise because they will always work better. However, supplements can work with them to raise your metabolic rate to even higher levels if you take the right ones.

The amino acid supplement known as Acetyl-L-Carnitine helps the body to naturally release growth hormones and enhances the function of the beta-oxidation process. This process is where the cells of your body burn fat for energy.

Hyaluronic Acid is a nutrient that helps repair the body's damaged cells and helps the body recover while you are sleeping. If you do a lot of exercise, you will also find this nutrient helps relieve lower back and joint pains as well. Then you will be able to sleep in comfort.

Vitamin C is an important vitamin that many people don't seem to consume. This vitamin helps the body recover and repair itself while you are sleeping. It also contains a number of antioxidants, and even promotes collagen synthesis.

Enjoying this book?

Check out my other best sellers!

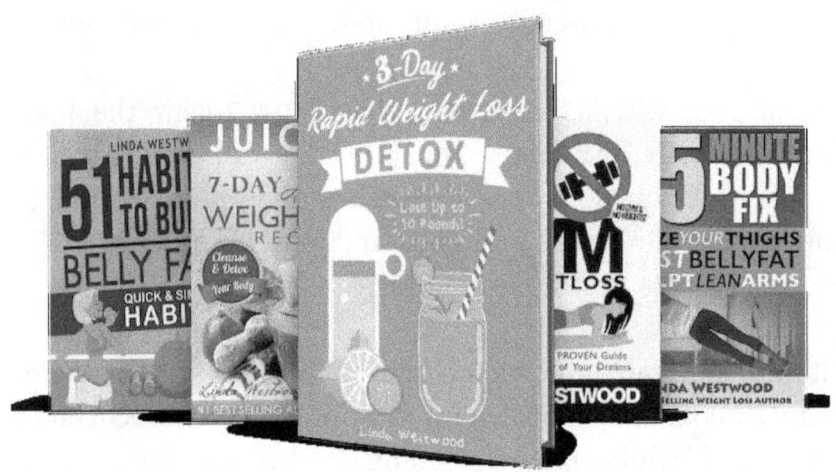

Get your next book on sale here:

TopFitnessAdvice.com/go/books

Step 6

Take Your Fat Burning to The Next Level

If you have made it this far then you already have enough discipline to take your fat burning to the next level. This is where you start an intermittent fasting regime. Fasting is when a person refrains from eating certain foods for a particular amount of time. With intermittent fasting, you are going to eat nothing for your first 14 to 20 hours. This means no calories whatsoever.

After 20 hours, you can eat as many calories as you need to boost your metabolism back up and lose weight. This will generally be about 1500 to 2000 calories within a short 4 to 10-hour timeframe. If you are trying to build muscle, then you will need over 2000 calories.

Now just continue this 24-hour fasting cycle with about 17 hours of no eating and then 7 hours of eating - until you burn the amount of fat that you wanted to burn. The best part is that you will continue to lose fat while you are asleep because your body will burn fat to produce energy and help your body recover for the next day.

Why it Works

Every time you finish a meal, the blood sugar and carbohydrates in your body rises. Your body burns these nutrients for energy, so that you can function. If you don't eat anything for extended periods of time, your carbohydrate and blood sugar levels will drop. Then your body will have to burn fat to produce energy instead of burning carbohydrates.

The built-up fat in people's bodies is just excess calories they consumed from overeating, which is why people get overweight in the first place.

Fasting allows the body to use those excess calories as sort of a backup energy supply. The result is less fat and a better appearance.

Make it Work for You

It might sound hard to go up to 20 hours without anything to eat. But remember that you also sleep for 8 hours as well. So you will only have 12 hours where you are awake and have to deal with your cravings.

When you are a beginner and first start intermittent fasting, your body will need some time to adjust to the change in your eating habits. That is why beginners should only go without eating for 12 hours instead of 20.

Therefore, if a beginner sleeps for 8 hours per day then they only have to worry about not eating for 4 hours while they are awake. These could be the 4 hours before they go to sleep, which will be the easiest to deal with because you have already had meals earlier in the day.

The side effects of fasting will vary between individuals. If you are somebody who has eaten junk foods without any discipline with dieting, then fasting may cause you to get headaches and dizziness because it will be such a new change to your body. If you feel physically sick or dizzy, you can break your fasting routine temporarily by eating a healthy snack that will get you feeling better again. Then go back to your fasting and complete the rest of the time you scheduled for yourself in the diet.

At an intermediate level, you will have successfully gone through a fasting regime and are accustomed to the changes it makes to your body. However, you may not be able to go 20 hours yet.

Intermediates simply need to work on increasing their fasting time as much as possible. This means going from 12 hours of fasting to about 16 hours. You can do this by refraining from eating for 8 hours before sleeping instead of 4 hours.

Then finally, experts who are comfortable with 16 hours of fasting can try for 20 hours and really jolt their system to the absolute limit. Just don't go over 20 hours because that will put your body into starvation mode, which is what you don't want.

Remember that intermittent fasting is not a lifestyle change that will last forever. You are only doing this to burn excess calories in a faster period of time. After you are done, you will want to go back to the six meals per day routine.

Additional Intermittent Fasting Tips

The idea behind intermittent fasting is that you do not consume any calories. However, you are technically allowed to consume beverages with no calories in it while you are fasting. This includes black coffee, green tea and water.

So, if you find yourself in the midst of a craving, drink plenty of calorie-free fluids to calm your hungry pains down.

Water is going to be your number one friend. Even though you are refraining from food for an extended period of time, you are not trying to dehydrate yourself in the process.

Your body depends on water more than it does food. Without water, you won't be able to survive. So, drink plenty of water and stay hydrated.

When you are ready to eat your meals, you will need to fit in a few thousand calories within a short 4-12-hour period. If it is a 4-hour period, then you should only have one big meal filled with lean meats, vegetables, fruits and whole grains.

This is referred to as the overeating phase, which advanced fasters will go through.

If you have up to 12 hours, you can have 3 meals split up over 4 hour intervals.

For the basic 2000-calorie requirement, try to consume 600-700 calories in each meal. This should be simple enough for people who are new to dieting and have already been accustomed to the basic 3 meal per day tradition.

If you work out at the gym most days during the week, then you have to make sure you eat a lot of carbohydrate filled foods before going to the gym.

If you are building muscle, then add protein rich foods to your meals as well. Then on your rest days, you should consume more fat than carbohydrates. Otherwise, you won't have any energy for the gym.

Once again, thank you for reading this book, and I hope you're getting a lot of valuable information. I would greatly appreciate it if you could take 30 seconds to leave me a review for this book on Amazon.com.

Step 7

Insulin Is Your Enemy

Insulin is a hormone that is responsible for regulating the sugar that gets absorbed by the cells of our body. We naturally produce insulin in our pancreas, but those who are diabetic or unable to produce insulin naturally will need to take it through medication.

The unfortunate side effect to taking insulin is the weight gain it will cause. Insulin allows glucose to absorb into your cells, which means your blood sugar level will decrease. So, if you consume too many calories while taking insulin, then your cells will become oversaturated with glucose and cause you to get fat as a result.

What you have to learn how to do is control your insulin levels by regulating and ultimately reducing them in order to effectively lose weight. There are a number of ways you can go about doing this.

Cutting Calories

People who take insulin for medical reasons truly have to watch their eating habits very carefully by counting every calorie they consume. The easiest way to go about this is to eat fewer calories in order to prevent weight gain.

Like always, consume only whole grains, vegetables, fruits and lean meats.

However, you have to measure all of your portions by studying the nutritional labels and determining the amount of calories and carbohydrates in your serving sizes for each meal.

For example, if you are on a 2000 calorie a day diet and eating 6 meals per day, then you need to consume 333 calories per meal. Any more calories while taking insulin will eventually get turned into fat.

Even though you are trying to cut calories, this doesn't mean skipping meals. If you skip a meal then your body won't produce as much energy, which means you will be extra hungry and likely make a poor eating choice. But worst of all, skipping meals will lower your blood sugar levels as well. If you are a diabetic trying to go on an intermittent fasting diet, then have a doctor help you with your nutritional plan.

Exercise

Physical exercise burns calories. This is another great way to regulate weight gain caused by increased insulin levels. But more importantly, it lowers blood glucose levels as well.

Insulin is very sensitive to exercise and intense physical activity. The cells of your body will be able to more effectively absorb glucose and turn it into energy, whether you have any insulin available or not.

If you are lifting weights and cause muscle contractions, this also allows your cells to absorb glucose and turn it into energy without need much insulin.

Therefore, you won't need to take as much insulin if you have a regular exercise routine that you follow.

Carbohydrate Cycling

You already know that carbohydrates are the main source of energy for the body. They help fuel your workouts and daily activities by increasing glucose levels in the body. But, what you may not realize is that carb cycling can actually help you lose fat and make you look the leanest you have ever been.

Carb cycling is where you alternate the amount of carbohydrates you intake per day. For example, you will have low carb days and high carb days which represent the amount of carbohydrate filled foods you will have in those days.

On your low carb days, you will still be eating carbs but you will only be eating clean carbs. This means you will only eat the amount of good carbs that you need to get through the day.

You can't be getting carbs from sugary foods and you can't eat any carb filled foods before going to sleep.

The reason eating carbohydrates is bad before bedtime is because your body doesn't need energy to function while it's asleep.

Therefore, it doesn't need to absorb carbohydrates for fuel. If you consume too many carbohydrates before bedtime, then it will get stored as fat in your body. This is what you don't want.

On your high carb days, you still want to eat clean carbs from food sources like whole grains, fruits and vegetables. However, this time you can eat more grams of carbohydrates per meal.

In a given high carb day, it is recommended that you consume 1 gram of carbs per pound of body weight. So, if you weigh 200 pounds, then you consume 200 grams of carbohydrates throughout the day.

The typical carb cycling routine is a pattern of 3 low carb days followed by 2 high carb days. Then you keep repeating the process until you have lost the necessary amount of weight.

When you first start the carb cycling process, you will want to keep reducing your normal carb intake by 50 grams on the low carb days.

Then you will increase the carbs by 75 grams when you go back to the high carb days. That way you won't shock your system too quickly. Instead, you will want to make it a gradual process.

For example, let's say your normal carb intake is 200 grams. You will make your first low carb day 150 grams, the second day 100 grams, and the third day 50 grams. Then when you start your high carb days, the first day will be 125 grams and the second day will be 200 grams.

The benefit to carb cycling is you will have less glucose getting absorbed in your cells, which results in producing less insulin in your pancreas.

That way, your cells won't become oversaturated with glucose and won't get stored as fat.

This is the result you want.

Get Some Sleep!

The most natural way to regulate insulin levels is to get a good night's sleep. This means getting your required 8 hours of rest without any tossing and turning, or going to the bathroom repeatedly.

Sleep stabilizes insulin levels, which means the cells of your body won't demand as much glucose. Then, they won't get stored as fat.

On top of that, if you have boosting your metabolic rate through the advice given in the previous steps, you will burn even more fat that is already stored in your body.

Step 8

Eat Junk Food & Lose Weight

Up until this point, there has been great emphasis put on eating healthy foods to lose weight. While this is a good thing to do, there are times when you can eat junk food. These times are called "cheat meals."

A cheat meal can be viewed in many different ways. For motivational purposes, cheat meals are often looked at as a reward for eating healthy after an extended period of time.

For example, a person may eat six healthy meals per day throughout the week.

Then on Saturday, they will indulge themselves in a meal that is not healthy.

Perhaps they will go out and have a cheeseburger or something else that is unhealthy in order to satisfy their junk food cravings.

This kind of behavior is great for losing weight, but you have to do it in moderation and not be too generous with your cheat meals.

The real point behind cheat meals is to regulate your addiction to the junk food that you have probably been accustomed to eating your whole life.

Junk foods, like soda, pizza, tacos, and candy, have salts and sugars that make them addictive.

In order to eat healthy, you have to beat the addiction. But like any addiction, you cannot just quit all together because you have to go through a withdrawal period. Cheat meals will be your way of getting through the withdrawal.

As you start to get used to healthy foods, the cheat meals will turn into a reward instead of a coping tactic. This reward system will become an incentive for you to continue on with your diet and not give up. Without this reward system, you may eventually decide to just give up your healthy way of living one day.

Keeping Your Metabolism Happy

It might be confusing to think of junk food actually boosting your metabolism because this book has already taught you the exact opposite. However, small amounts of junk food incorporated into your life per week will still allow you to burn fat.

The first thing you have to remember is never have multiple cheat meals throughout the course of a day. You should only have a cheat meal once per day, with the rest of the meals being healthy.

Your cheat meal should never be the first meal of the day. Instead, it should be one of the last. That way you can keep your metabolic rate high throughout the day.

Then your metabolism won't be so dependent on the empty calories you will be consuming from your cheat meal.

Make sure the rest of your earlier meals are smaller healthy meals, like previously discussed. You can cut 100 calories or so from these meals on the day you plan to have your cheat meal. Only consume the minimum amount of healthy calories you need for energy. This will make up for the excess junk calories you will be consuming later on.

Whatever you do, do not fast leading up to your cheat meal. Some people think if they eliminate all calories until their cheat meal, that it will keep them thin.

But, all this will do is make your metabolism more dependent on the empty calories and carbohydrates from the cheat meal.

Don't Go Crazy

If you are first starting out with a diet plan, it is best to have a nutritionist or personal trainer write your meal plan for you. That way they can decide how often you should have your cheat meals.

Typically, cheat meals are not supposed to be eaten more than 1-2 times per week. But if you are severely obese, then your trainer may let you have a cheat meal every other day instead. That way it does not shock your system too much when you try to change your diet.

As time goes on, you will gradually move away from eating cheat meals every other day and then allow yourself just one day a week for the cheat meal. This is where you want to be.

Of course, you can still make mistakes with your one cheat meal if you don't know what you are doing. For one thing, you need to keep the size of your cheat meal within reason.

No one expects you to count calories in your cheat meal, but it doesn't mean you can go pig out at the nearest Chinese buffet either. If anything, try to keep the portion size of your cheat meal equal to the portion size of your healthy meals. At least that way the density of the calories and nutrients will be the same.

The worst thing you can do is pig out in your cheat meal because then you won't be hungry for any more meals. Not only that, but it will make it harder for you to get to sleep as well.

You have already learned that a good night's sleep is important for your metabolism levels to stay high and burn fat. So make sure your cheat meal isn't big enough to give you stomach cramps and gas all night long.

If you follow the advice from this chapter and eat your cheat meals in moderation, then it will not affect your weight loss goals whatsoever. Instead, they will help you stick to your goals and not give up on them.

Step 9

Boost Your Fat Burning TODAY!

The final step to burning fat while you sleep is taking supplements to further boost your metabolic rate.

We have already covered this briefly in the book, but you need to understand the many different types of supplements and brands that are available on the market.

How Supplements Burn Fat

Do not misunderstand what the power of supplements. They are not some quickie fix to losing weight.

They are not magical pills that will burn away all your fat and give you six-pack abs. These kinds of pills do not exist, so don't ever solely rely on supplements to lose weight.

Supplements should be thought of an assistant to your metabolism. They can help push a high metabolic rate even higher. That is what you need to understand about them.

Types of Supplements

Now there are different types of supplements that have their own way of boosting your metabolism. One way is through **genetic engineering**. There is an antioxidant called Sesamin, which is derived from sesame oil.

Sesamin is not only a powerful antioxidant, but it is a great fat burner. It turns on certain receptors in the cells of your heart, muscle and liver that is called PPAR Alpha. Once these receptors become activated, they will activate your fat burning genes by reducing the amount of fat stored in your body.

Another genetic supplement is tetradecylthioacetic acid, or TTA.

This is a fatty acid that does not get burned by the body, while still being able to regular the storage and burning of other dietary fats. It can also help reduce insulin sensitivity, which means you won't need as much insulin as normal to absorb glucose.

Mineral supplements, such as selenium, zinc and calcium, can help you prevent fat gain and even assist with fat loss.

If you take a multivitamin then it may have a small percentage of these minerals in it, but you may need more. Your daily value of these minerals has to be 100%, so watch your nutritional charts carefully.

Calcium is responsible for regulating a hormone called calcitriol, which is what assists the body in producing fat in the first place.

When calcium levels are high, calcitriol is controlled. It also allows your intestines to absorb less dietary fat, which will result in fat loss as well.

Zinc promotes the production of thyroid hormones, which will increase your metabolic rate. People who are low in zinc will have a low metabolic rate. So, you will want to make sure you get enough zinc through a supplement source.

Selenium is another mineral that is needed for the production of thyroid hormones. Without selenium, your metabolic rate will also suffer as a result.

With calcium and selenium supplements, they should be taken with food once per day. The calcium dosage should be about 1,000 mg and the selenium should be 300 mcg.

As for the zinc, this absorbs better on an empty stomach. That is why it is recommended to take zinc before going to sleep. All you need is 30 mg of it, and your metabolic rate will be high throughout the night.

Finally, **amino acid supplements** have fat burning qualities to them. As you may know, amino acids are found in protein and allow the muscles to absorb them for growth.

What many people don't realize is that a few amino acids have fat burning properties to them as well. These amino acids are arginine and glutamine. Glutamine is an amino acid that increases the body's metabolic rate and fat burning properties. It does this by increasing lipolysis in the body, which frees up fat from existing fat cells. If you are a weight lifter then you will probably find glutamine in many protein powders that are out on the market.

Arginine is an amino acid that boosts the nitric oxide levels in your body, but it also doubles as a fat burner. It does this by also increasing lipolysis in your body. What fat is freed from fat cells through this process, it becomes much easier for the body to burn the fat and turn it into fuel.

Glutamine and arginine should be taken together for best results.

The recommended glutamine dosage is 5-10 grams with breakfast or before working out.

The recommended arginine dosage is 3-10 grams, but it should be taken before breakfast or 60 minutes before exercising. You should also take arginine after workouts and 60 minutes before going to bed as well.

The Right Time to Take Supplements

There is a reason why supplement consumption is the final step to this 9-step system. The reason is because you want to go through all of the other steps that involve healthy eating, small portion meals and exercise because they are the most important parts of boosting your metabolism.

Supplements should only be taken when you reach a plateau in your weight loss goals. This is a point where you still want to lose more weight, but you just don't see the results taking place even though you are putting in the right amount of effort.

Plateaus often happen when your body becomes accustomed to the same routine over and over again. That is why people will tell you to trick your body when it comes to diet and exercise.

Changing your routines will always create a new outcome when trying to lose weight.

Supplements can be helpful because they will allow you to stick to your routine while making changes to your metabolism in the process.

Others who are considering purchasing this book would love to know what you think. If you could spare a few seconds, they would greatly appreciate reading an honest review from you. Simply view the page on Amazon.com.

Don't Forget This!

You have now learned the 9 steps to losing weight while you sleep. The important thing to remember is to follow these steps in chronological order for the best results in burning fat during your sleeping periods.

The 9-step system is not just a bunch of weight loss tips. Sure, some of these steps could be used independently in other types of weight loss programs, but your focus here is to try to lose weight while you sleep.

This can only be done by going through the steps featured in this book, from beginning to end. There are no shortcuts here.

The whole philosophy behind this 9-step system is to boost your metabolic rate, so that way you can sleep and burn fat at the same time.

You will never find a pill or infomercial gadget on television that will successfully do this solely for you. Instead you have to implement real world solutions to boost your metabolic rate by eating right and exercising.

As you learned in the 9th step, you can add supplements to your routine once you have conquered all the other harder steps that require you to diet and exercise.

Do not ever depend on supplements alone because they require you to assist them by making healthy choices in your life.

If you are an absolute beginner then you may lag on a few of these steps, but do not give up!

The worst thing you can ever do is give up because you think you cannot do it. This system is not meant to be a walk in the park. It is going to be difficult and requires you to really want to lose weight in order to succeed.

The only time fat burning is easy is when you are asleep because your body does all the work. However, you have to work to get your body in a position to where it can actually make you lose weight while you sleep.

As you know, this means boosting your metabolic rate which is where the difficulty comes into play.

Do not worry because the system gets easier as time goes on and you get more disciplined. It is similar to how somebody who lifts weights for the first time feels sore in their muscles. But after a while, they won't feel as sore anymore. Just develop this kind of mentality and you will get through these steps with no problems.

By implementing the 9-step system into your daily life to boost your metabolic rate, you will burn fat, lose weight and ultimately change your life forever.

Thank you for reading this book. I hope you found it educational and inspiring at the same time. Please leave me some positive feedback when you get a chance and let me know if the information helped you.

The PROVEN & EFFECTIVE Way to Boost Your Metabolism Permanently

What You Will Learn Next

If you are looking to lose weight in a fast and safe way, you should first try and understand your metabolism. The metabolism rate of your body determines the amounts of fats and carbs that are burned for energy in your body. In this eBook, you will learn about how to increase the metabolism rate of your body to increase the amounts of fats burned in your body.

You will also learn about many other methods of weight loss tips and even some of the recipes that are good for you as you work on your weight. Losing weight tips are some of the most sort after tips in an age where being fat is seen as a disease. This eBook will provide you with simple to execute ideas on how you can get rid of the extra pounds.

The recipes included are some of the most delicious but still very healthy dishes that you can be consuming. They are packed with enough energy to keep you going and also to help in the improvement of your metabolism rate.

Understanding Your Metabolism

If you are serious about losing those extra pounds that you have on your body, you should first try and understand your metabolism and how it is working. Most people end up not losing weight after working out and even cutting down on calories just because they do not understand their metabolisms functionality.

Poor metabolism can result in you maintaining that unhealthy shape even if you frequent the gym. This means that you are suffering from low metabolism and for your health to improve you will have to do something about that.

Exercise and proper dieting can help you in improving your metabolism rate if used properly. You should make sure you understand your metabolism thoroughly so that you are able to come up with a good combination of dishes that will help.

Metabolism can be defined as the chemical processes in which a body burns up fats that are unwanted in the body and are found lodged in the body. It is used to give the body energy to be able to carry out tasks that are important to you. The speed of the metabolism rate will be affected by any exercise that you do in and out of the gym.

The most basic and minimum amount of energy a body requires to carry out a task also known as basal metabolic rate takes up between forty and seventy of the daily generated energy by your body. The amount of energy use will depend mainly on your lifestyle and age.

We get energy and strength from the breaking down of fats, this enables us to move around, think and do many other things. We also try to burn more fats using energy generated from other fats.

Factors That Determine Your Metabolic Rate

There are a few factors that determine the rate of your metabolism also known as the basal metabolic rate. The great news is that no matter how low your basal metabolic rate gets, you can easily improve it. The most basic factors that you will have to worry about will include some of the following:

Body Size

Most fat people always tend to blame the metabolism rate for their bodies accumulating fats. You might think that your huge body is the reason that your metabolism is low, but the truth is that a huge body requires lots of energy and thus your basal metabolic rate will have been high. Even with the fact that the people with big bodies burn more fats for energy, you might wonder why they remain huge.

For a fat person, the most common reason as to why they are not able to lose weight through metabolism is because they are consuming more calories than they are burning up. With there being extra calories in the body, it is forced to store them up for use in the future.

If you are huge and you want to lose massive amounts of weight in a short period of time, you should start by reducing your intake and increasing the basal metabolic rate of your body. You should also work on gaining muscles because it has been proven that muscle cells will use up more energy than the fat cells. Therefore, fat people will have a lower basal metabolic rate than a muscular person.

Age

As you grow old you will reach a certain point where your basal metabolic rate starts to decrease after every ten years. Age leads the human body into losing muscles and gain more fats thus resulting to decreased metabolic rates. You will also happen to lose lean muscles which should be retained at all costs. To ensure that you do not start storing unwanted calories due to the reduced rate of metabolism, you should decrease the intake of your calories respectively.

You could also become more active in the sense of exercising. Exercising is one of the most successful way of burning lots of calories.

Gender

In both genders the rate of metabolism in the body goes down with age but it is slower in men than among the women. The male species tends to always have more muscles, heavier bones and less body fat than the females and this hugely contributes to why men have both high calories intake and metabolism rates.

Genes

If you take an adopted child, you will find that he or she will have physical features of the biological parents and not the ones that brought him up. This goes to show that genes do somehow contribute to whether one will have a low or high metabolism rate before any exercise or activities.

They have been suspected to contribute to deciding the basic rate of each human's rate of metabolic in their bodies, though this has not been proved to be a sure thing and also as how it functions.

A Sample Diet & Recipe

When you are taking this eBook as a guide to your weight loss, there are certain types of foods that you will need to be taking in your first section of the process. These foods are ones that will help you with your metabolism and also allow your body to burn and not store fats.

In this section, the food that you eat for breakfast should contain fruit and grain; your midday snack should be a fruit. At lunch time, you should make sure that your meal consists of grain, fruit, vegetables and proteins.

Your evening snack should be a fruit too and for dinner you should have grains, vegetables and proteins. The idea here is to keep the amount of food consumed at a high level but with the ability of increasing your metabolism's rate. This will in return lead to better health and the use of all fats for energy thus leading to fast and safe weight loss.

One of the foods that you can cook that contains grains includes food such as the oatmeal pancakes. The following is the recipe of oatmeal pancakes that you can easily use to cook some at home.

Sample Recipe: Oatmeal Pancakes

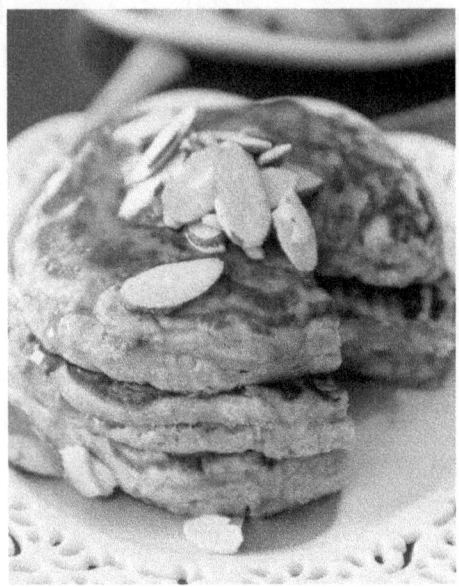

The preparation of oatmeal pancakes will require you to have all of the following ingredients and in the given sizes.

Ingredients

Serves: 8
Yields: 16 four-inch pancakes

- 2 cups nonfat milk
- 1 teaspoon of vanilla extract
- 3 cups rolled oats
- 2 lightly beaten eggs

- 1 teaspoon baking powder
- 1 teaspoon ground cinnamon

Directions

1. Take the oats and blend them for sixty seconds to a fine flour consistency.

2. Take the powder and put it in a big bowl, then take cinnamon, salt and the baking powder and add them into the bowl and mix thoroughly.

3. Take the vanilla extract and mix it in a small bowl together with the eggs and milk.

4. Take both the dry and liquid mixtures and mix them together till they are just moist. Now leave the mixture to rest for about five minutes.

5. Using medium heat, take a nonstick skillet and place it over the fire and once it gets hot you can pour a quarter cup of batter for a pancake.

6. Let the pancake cook until there are bubbles on the surface, then turn it over and cook the other side to a light brown.

I hope you have learned something from this book so far and would greatly appreciate it if you could leave an honest review on Amazon.com.

Fat Burning and Body Toning Foods

When it comes to losing weight the right way and by the method involving your metabolism, you will find that there are foods that will help you in losing weight. These foods also happen to help with the composition of a great body physique. They mainly contain huge amounts of proteins, carbs and healthy fats which are essential for a lean body and its maintenance. They also help you feel energized all day long. The foods that you should consume in this category include the following:

Eggs

The proteins in an egg contain sufficient amounts of choline which prevents the liver from accumulating fats and also protects it.

Choline is also a predecessor of an energizing neurotransmitter which is called an acetylcholine. If increased, acetylcholine leads to the raised point of growth hormones. These hormones happen to be very powerful fat burners. Through their thermic effects, eggs will give you a nice metabolism boost as a result of their elevated protein content.

The cholesterol in the eggs is to improve the authenticity of the muscle cell membranes and to produce testosterone. The cholesterol does not increase or trigger the increment of serum cholesterol.

In this section, you should be consuming at least two eggs a day. This will help in increasing the levels of protein and choline intake in your body.

Coffee

There are no any conclusive results of a study on the benefits or role played by coffee in burning a lot of calories by the metabolism process. Coffee also helps the body focus on fats rather than glucose as a source of energy. It also helps the body against oxygen species that are harmful, helps modulate the blood and also minimizes the risk of Alzheimer's disease.

It is estimated that drinking of five hundred milliliters of coffee daily could help an overweight person lose about five pounds.

If you are looking for improved performance caused by the boosting and motivating your energy, caffeinated coffee is what you should be taking. Drinking of caffeinated coffee right before working out will help you go the extra mile and even increase your workout intensity.

A healthy diet and proper intense workouts accompanied by a good cup of caffeinated coffee will help you again and maintain a great body composition. You will also be able to lose huge amounts of fats in the process.

Berries

To ensure that you have a healthy and well-formed body, you should make sure that you have one serving of berries at the very least each day. You can also mix them with fruits such as pomegranate and mangoes to make the dish more interesting. Consumption of the same dish prepared in the same way gets boring over time and may make you lose interest in eating healthy.

The berries that you should be going for include strawberries, blueberries and raspberries. These berries contain antioxidant and this makes them very good for the burning of fats. They also contain fiber and are also blunt to insulin. Foods with high carbohydrates result to the body producing huge amounts of insulin.

The sensitivity of the brain to leptin causes someone to not feel that much hungry, all this is caused by antioxidants known as Ellagitannins found in raspberries.

Vegetables and Broccoli Cruciferous

If you have any estrogen in your body, whether it occurred naturally or chemically, you can be able to get rid of it by making sure that you consume your vegetables. Vegetables such as broccoli and cauliflower will help you make sure that you eliminate any unwanted estrogen in your body.

Vegetables contain compounds that make them able to interact with the estrogen binding genes. This is what makes vegetables good for a person in the pursuit of weight loss.

The vegetables contain high fiber which they use to favorably change the response of the body to glucose. This happens as a result of delayed absorption of carbohydrates. The high fiber in vegetables can also play a vital role of restraining the insulin response; this makes them the best food for someone looking to lose weight.

You will also gain lots of antioxidants from the consumption of green vegetables. It is wise that you consume them raw for maximum gains, but you can cook them if you are not okay with raw vegetables. Have at least a couple of servings a day, every day.

Avocados

A single avocado fruit contains quite a number of beneficial things such as 15 grams of healthy fats, about two hundred and fifty calories, proteins 4 grams, fiber 10 grams and twenty vital nutrients.

Avocados contain remarkable antioxidants and this makes it a very strong anti-obesity fruit to consume.

Nuts

Nuts such as almonds and walnuts are quite high in antioxidant healthy fats, proteins and fibers. Consuming them would result in the body losing unwanted weight. You can go ahead and add them to your meals and they will assist in giving you an improved body composition.

The consumption of nuts will not only boost your metabolic response but also boost feelings of blunt appetite and satiety.

For the best results, it is advisable that you consume walnuts with their skin, this makes them very healthy and they contain high levels of antioxidants.

For any elimination of waste from the body, you should make sure that you consume almonds. Almonds are high in vitamin E, fiber and protein making them suitable for the elimination of waste from the body.

Make sure that you at least consume these nuts once in a day and you will be always feel satisfied and be able to lose fats.

Cold Water Fish

Whitefish, sardines, anchovies, mackerel and salmon are some of the examples of cold water fish. These cold water fish contain high omega-3 unsaturated fats. Inflammation and the improvement of insulin sensitivity can be taken care of by the use of omega-3 fats.

Once the sensitivity of your insulin is increased, it will help your body not to store the carbs in form of fats but as muscles glycogen.

With reduced inflammation, you are able to enjoy food more and also metabolic hormones will be balanced leading to reduced feelings of hunger and having a high metabolism rate. The less you eat will be a lot satisfying and will be put to good use.

Research shows that if you consume about 4 grams of omega-3 for about forty-five days, you will have reduced the amount of fats in your body and gained some lean mass too. This is something that was carried out under observation to see if the results would be true, and they were.

Vinegar

If you want to make sure that whenever you eat your body stores the carbohydrates inform of muscle glycogen and not as fats, you should make the use of vinegar a habit. Consumption of vinegar in your meals will improve the functions of your pancreas and lowers your insulin to carbs.

For a moderated elevation of your blood sugar and many more benefits from vinegar, just add some to your salad and you will reap all the benefits that are there in it.

The best and sweet tasting vinegars in the market are the balsamic and white wine vinegar, but any kind of vinegar that you use will still give you these great benefits and even help in losing of fat.

These foods that have been elaborated above will be very helpful to you on your journey to lose weight. These foods will do the following in your body in line with helping you to lose weight:

I. Basically, they will make your body rely more on fats for energy and not on carbohydrates; this way you will be able to get rid of the fats and still feel energized all day.

II. They decrease the levels of inflammation and improve the sensitivity of insulin in your cells. They also make sure that your body uses the blood sugar in the carbohydrates to generate energy for usage in the body.

III. By increasing the metabolism rate of a resting body, this will lead to the burning down of more fats for energy. They will help in the repairing of tissues so that you keep burning down more energy.

IV. Increasing leptin to blunt the hunger feelings, elimination of excess estrogen, lowering of insulin and cortisol- all which is done through the improvement of hormones response to food.

Tips on How to Speed Up Your Basal Metabolic Rate

The basal metabolic rate is the speed at which your body burns and breaks down fats for energy. If you have a very low metabolism rate you can easily increase it to make it work faster and burn more fats to lose more weight.

There are workouts and diets that you can use to make sure that your metabolism is always working at full capacity. This will help you shed off extra pounds of fats in your body that you really do not need.

Working out and watching what you eat will increase your basal metabolic rate to about 600 calories a day.

If you are looking to lose fats that are not good for you, just make sure that you get the workouts in line with your body. This will maximize the level at which you will be burning fats.

Some Tips to Speed Up Your Metabolism

The tips that are provided below have been designed to guide you improve your basal metabolic rate and help you lose as much fat as possible. They include the following:

- **Consume more foods that are rich in fiber and protein**

    Digesting of foods with lots of proteins and are high in fibers will elevate the resting metabolism rate of your body.

    So, the more of these foods that you consume, the better your metabolism becomes and it even gets more comfortable. Ensure that the foods have lots of complex carbs and are at least thirty percent proteins.

- **The After Burn**

    This is the ability of a body to keep on burning fats even long after you are done working out. The intensity of your exercise will help you lose more calories and even enable the burning of the fats to go on after you leave the gym.

    For the best after burn effect you should do some high intensity interval training every other day. Once you do some of these workouts, your body will be burning calories for a couple of days. This results to losing more weight and in no time at all.

- **Thyroid Function**

    When your body lacks nutrients, your metabolism will automatically slow down. When your metabolism is slow, you risk the chance of developing hypothyroidism.

The thyroid gland is a regulator of your body's metabolism and its functionality can be boosted by the consumption of foods that are rich in zinc, selenium, iodine, copper and vitamin E, basically nuts and seafood.

- **Drinking Lots of Water**

For a person who is looking to lose weight, it is wise that you make sure to drink a liter of water each day at the very least. Water will help you increase the basal metabolic rate of your body and also keep you from bloating.

The colder the water that you drink, the better for your body for it will boost the rate of your metabolism with the aim of producing more energy to get and keep you warm. It will also help in flushing out excess water weight from your body.

It has been proven through research and studies, that ten minutes after you drink cold water, your basal metabolic rate is increased by a staggering thirty percent.

- **Going With no Breakfast**

When you wake up in the morning your body requires energy to face the day, if you skip your breakfast, your body will be forced to look elsewhere for the energy.

This leaves the body with no choice but to burn more fats for energy that you need to get through the day.

Breakfast might be the most important meal of the day, and in skipping it you might actually stand a better chance of weight loss.

- **Boost Your Human Growth Hormone**

   The human growth hormone is the one that helps your body to build up on muscles and also helps in maintaining them.

   A lot of energy is needed for this process and that results to an increased rate of metabolism in your body.

   If you can manage to boost the levels of human growth hormone in your body, you will end up using more energy meaning high metabolic rates and the burning of more calories and fats.

- **Morning Workouts**

   Morning workouts are the best option for people looking to shed off some extra pounds. Like many things, the way that you start up your metabolism for the day matters a lot.

   Morning exercise will help you start a day with a high metabolism and also help in the maintaining of that rate. You can always wake early and work on some intense exercise and you will be in a great position of burning calories all day long. This will help with the quick loss of fats that you are looking for.

Evening workouts on the other hand are not as reliable and useful, once you build up a metabolism and you are just about to go to bed, it will not take long for the rate to slow down.

This is because once you go to bed and your body has nothing to do but rest. Try and squeeze in your workouts in the morning.

- **Work on Gaining Muscle**

    The more muscles that you have in your body will enable you to burn more calories through metabolism. With every muscles pound, you will burn a maximum of twelve calories in a day.

    The simple math is that, the more the muscles you have, the higher the number of burned calories.

    With that, you can see the importance of working on gaining more muscles as you are working on losing weight. For any exercise that you do, you will end up using more calories since your muscles will all require energy as you work out.

- **Keeping Active**

    No matter what you are doing, your body will always be burning fats or carbs for energy. Keeping busy is another way of ensuring that you are losing fats and that your basal metabolic rate is not basic.

You can start by walking to work or the mall if you do not live so far from both places. Avoid taking the bus unless it is very necessary, like if you live far from your work place or if you leave work at a late hour for an evening walk.

- **Using Spices**

Consumption of spices has been studied and found to boost the basal metabolic rate of a body by up to twenty percent. This effect can last for up to thirty minutes depending on the spices used.

You just have to add some pepper of any other form of spices in your meal and eat it. The hotness of the spices will lead to increased metabolism rates for a given period of time. You will burn a little more fat this way.

- **Caffeine Consumption**

Consumption of between fifty and three hundred milliliters of coffee is seen as the moderate volume and it can easily increase the resting metabolism rate of your body. Caffeine also boosts the rate at which metabolism takes place by producing adrenaline.

When you drink coffee just before you start working out, it helps in increasing the number of fats that you will end up burning during your workout session.

Keep in mind that whatever exercise that you do will have some sort of after burn. It might not be much as that of the high intensity workouts, but it helps a bit.

High intensity training is the only form of exercise that will leave your body burning fats long after you are done working out.

Make you workouts last for about ten minutes and do them during the day. These small interval intense workouts are the best and are more helpful than taking the long ones.

Sample Diet

In this section, you should make sure that your daily meal consists of the following foods.

Breakfast, lunch, dinner and your snacks should consist of proteins and vegetables. Make sure that the vegetables and proteins differ for each meal so that you have some sort of variety.

Proteins could include anything from white egg, smoked salmon, tuna, turkey jerky and strip steak among many others. For veggies, you can have either spinach, cucumbers, red pepper and steamed broccoli among other vegetables.

Sample Recipe: Chicken and Brown Rice Soup

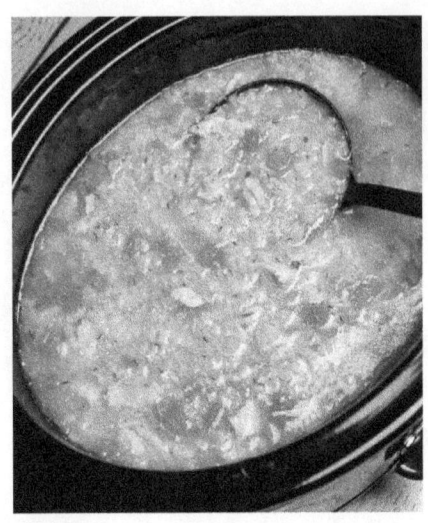

Serves: 4

Ingredients

- 4 cups low-sodium chicken broth, divided
- 1/2 chopped medium onion
- 1 1/2 chopped medium carrots
- 1 stalk celery, chopped
- 1 cup water
- 1/2 cup long-grain brown rice
- 1 small chicken breast, cut into 1/4-inch cubes
- 1/2 bay leaf
- 1/2 bunch kale, thinly sliced leaves

Directions

1. Take a large pot and bring half a cup of broth to simmer at over medium-high heat.

2. Then add carrots, celery and onion and cook for about 8 minutes, stirring occasionally.

3. Take the remaining 3 1/2 cups broth, rice, water, bay leaf and chicken and boil them.

4. Then reduce the heat down to a simmer, cover and cook for about half an hour or until the chicken is cooked or the rice becomes tender.

5. Remove the bay leaf and stir in kale. You should continue cooking till the kale is wilted and tender, it will take about three to five minutes.

Nutrition

When you are planning on losing weight, you will find out that exercise is not all there is to it. What you eat and drink also matters a lot.

Proper nutrition will enable you to be able to come up with a system that will help you burn those nagging fats and also help you maintain the muscles you have.

Eating more foods that are high in proteins and fiber is a good strategy of weight loss, going on some crazy diet or starting one of those programs where you have to calculate every calorie you eat will lead to the reduction of your basal metabolic rate.

If your body does not find the calories to burn, it will then turn to your muscles for energy.

So, the more you take those crashed diets, the more you will keep subjecting your body to feeding off your muscles. Once you stop the diet program, you will build back up the fats that you were getting rid of since your metabolism rate will have decreased during the diet.

Avoid these diets and take a much better way that will leave you with your muscles and no fats even after you have stopped working out for some time.

There are meals that you should take before and after you work out, the following subheading will be focusing on the nutrition tips that will help you after you are done working out.

Post-Workout Nutrition Tips

One of the most important foods for someone who is looking to lose weight is the proteins. You should know that what you consume matters a lot when it comes to the amount of weight that you have lost and what your target is.

Working out all the time is not necessarily the best way to go if you want to lose weight. With proper nutrition, you will be able to maintain and even gain new muscles, you will also be able to lose weight the right way without torturing yourself.

As you work out and look for the best food for your body, you should at least consume food with about 25 grams of proteins. Out of the twenty-five grams, ten should have come from vital amino acids. Forty percent of the ten grams comes from a branched amino acid known as leucine.

One needs to keep the muscle protein synthesis high at all times and this is will require that you ingest huge amounts of proteins.

Using of proteins and proper workout produces a synergistic effect and you should make sure that you always take the proteins after you are done working out. This is because the building of muscles is mainly activated through some intense contractions of your already existing muscles.

Milk protein is superior than that of food even soy, leucine which is found in milk, is big on protein synthesizing. It can do so for about twenty-four hours.

Older people should consume large quantities of proteins for it is great for their health; this is yet to be proven.

Whey Proteins

These are found to be more superior than all the other forms of proteins, this is as a result of their fast digestion in your body and they also containing leucine. This compound is hypertrophy to senior citizens, men and women. Whey proteins can greatly help in the improvement of muscles building to both an individual or a given physiological situations.

The following are some of the ways that you can use when you are taking your proteins. These ways have been devised so that you may be able to take your proteins for maximum benefits. They include the following:

Consumption of some proteins just before going to bed will help you with your overnight protein synthesis.

Consuming some whey proteins after your work out can act as a very good source of nutrients. Ensure that you do consume some whenever you work out.

The most constructive dose of protein in grams per kilogram of your body weight should be 0.25 grams and 0.3 kilograms.

Make sure that they are the best proteins in every meal that you consume.

Taking of large doses of leucine in every meal that you consume will play a big role in the prediction of whether there is any post meal protein fusion response.

Ensure that for every kilogram of your body weight, you consume at least 1.6 grams of proteins. This will help with make sure that the fat loss process happens quickly.

Don't forget to share your thoughts on this book by leaving a review on Amazon.com. It takes just a few seconds.

Factors That May Slow Down Metabolism

The rate of your metabolism cannot only be accelerated, but there are some ways that may cause it to slow down –which is not a good thing.

Your body's metabolism can be slowed down by quite a number of conditions and even diseases. Some of the illnesses that you should watch out for include Cushing's syndrome and hypothyroidism.

Your lifestyle too could be causing you to gain pounds of extra fats and it would be nice if you were to visit a doctor and get some advice on healthy living.

Other factors that can affect your metabolism include:

- **Excess Alcohol**

    Consumption of alcohol will also cause your metabolism to slow down by a staggering seventy three percent. This will remain so for more than a couple hours. Alcohol also gives you extra weight since it contains empty calories.

- **Skipping Meals**

    Though skipping of meals can be interpreted as a good thing since you are cutting down on calories, skipping meals puts a break on your metabolism.

Your body requires a certain number of calories for it to function properly in a day, the problem is that most people take this to a whole new level and end up starving their bodies.

- **Caffeine**

Caffeine is good for you when you take it in qualities that are well regulated; it increases the rate of your body's metabolism. The problem comes in when you start to over use it. It can have some undesired effects such as but not limited to:

- Rapid Heart Rates
- Frequent Urination
- Lack of Sleep
- Headaches
- Nausea
- Muscles Tremors
- Anxiety

Sample Diet

In this last section of the diet you should be having a meal that is more about ensuring that your metabolism keeps working properly as you have guided it so far.

In your meals, make sure that your breakfast is made up of a fruit, egg's fat, vegetables and grains, your snacks should have some hummus fat and vegetables.

For lunch, have some proteins, vegetables and healthy fats (avocado), for snacks have some vegetables and a little fat. For dinner, you should have some grains, vegetables and proteins.

Sample Recipe: Italian Style Penne (Slow Cooker)

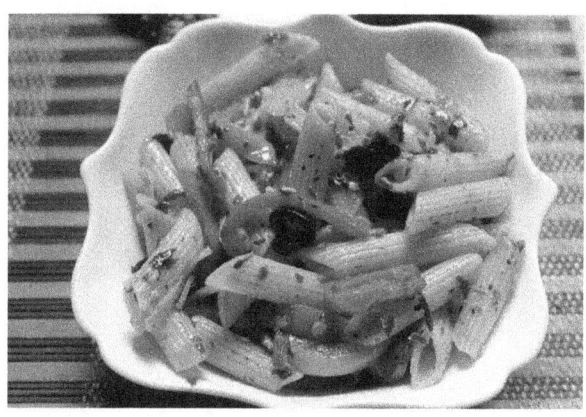

Yields: 6 servings

Ingredients

- 2 cans of diced tomatoes that are low on sodium
- 1/2 pound dry, whole wheat penne pasta
- 1 tablespoon seasoning, Italian herb
- 1 tablespoon grounded garlic
- 1/2 cup low sodium, chicken or vegetable broth
- 1 can of kidney beans, drained and rinsed
- Balsamic Vinegar
- 1 tablespoon powdered onion
- Parmesan cheese for garnish

Directions

1. After you have warmed up your slow cooker, lay your ingredients one after the other. Start by placing your penne pasta at the bottom, followed by your diced tomatoes.

2. You should then add the kidney beans and then pour over the vegetable broth on top.

3. Then sprinkle the onions, Italian seasoning herbs and garlic over the dish.

4. Let it cook for about one to two hours or till the pasta is cooked and finally add some balsamic vinegar for taste.

5. You should then cover the top of the readymade dish with some fresh grated cheese.

Discover Scientifically-Proven "Shortcuts" & "Hacks" to Lose Weight FASTER (With Very Little Effort)

For this month only, you can get Linda's best-selling & most popular book absolutely free – *Weight Loss Secrets You NEED to Know*.

Get Your FREE Copy Here:
TopFitnessAdvice.com/Bonus

Discover scientifically-proven tips to help you lose weight faster and easier than ever before. With this book, readers were able to improve their weight loss results and fitness levels. So, it's highly recommended that you get this book, especially while it's free!

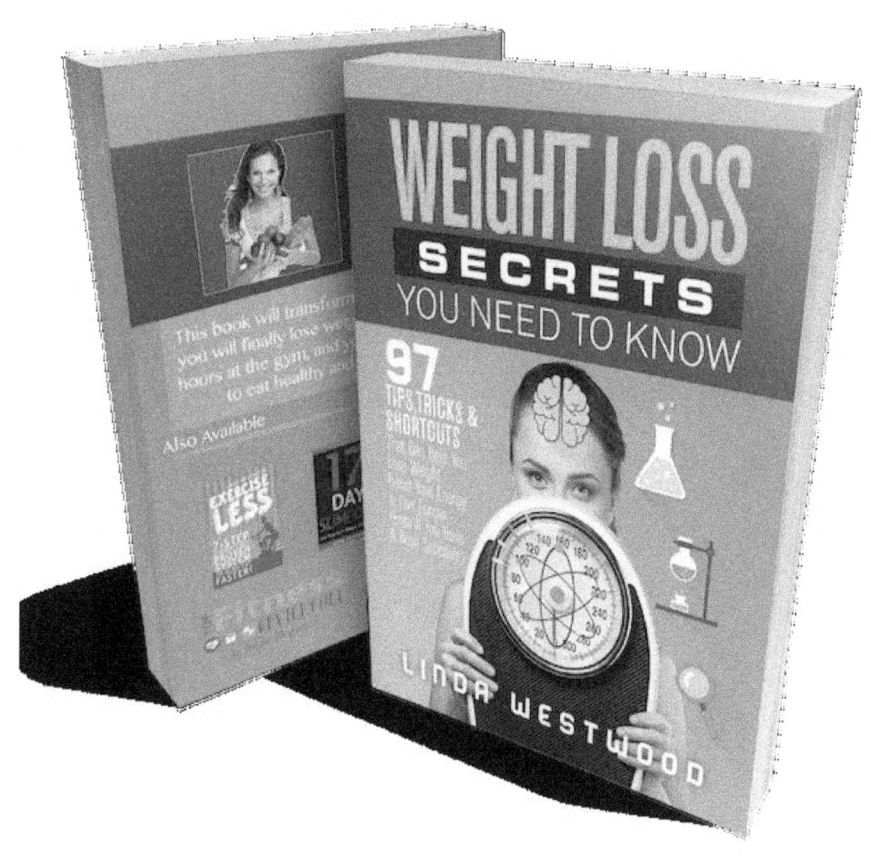

Get Your FREE Copy Here:

TopFitnessAdvice.com/Bonus

Final Words

I would like to thank you for purchasing my book and I hope I have been able to help you and educate you on something new.

If you have enjoyed this book and would like to share your positive thoughts, could you please take 30 seconds of your time to go back and give me a review on my Amazon book page.

I greatly appreciate seeing these reviews because it helps me share my hard work.

You can leave me a review on Amazon.com.

Again, thank you and I wish you all the best!

Enjoying this book?

Check out my other best sellers!

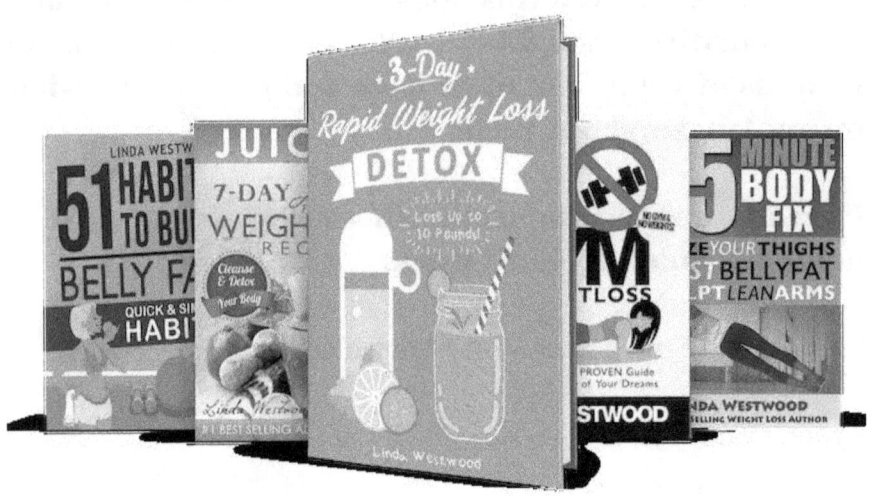

Get your next book on sale here:

TopFitnessAdvice.com/go/books

www.ingramcontent.com/pod-product-compliance
Lightning Source LLC
Chambersburg PA
CBHW031158020426
42333CB00013B/723